Natural Antibiotics

Natural Homemade Remedies to Prevent, Heal and Cure Common Illnesses, Infections and Allergies

Disciaimer

Although the author and publisher have made every effort to ensure that the information in this book was correct at press time, the author and publisher do not assume and hereby disclaim any liability to any party for any loss, injury, damage or disruption caused by errors or omissions, whether such errors or omissions result from negligence, accident, non-functional websites, or any other cause. Any advice or strategy contained herein may not be suitable for every individual. Information in this book should not be used as a substitute for professional medical prevention, diagnosis, or treatment. Please consult with your physician, pharmacist, or health care provider before taking any home remedies or supplements or following any treatment suggested. Only your health care provider, personal physician, or pharmacist can provide you with advice on what is safe and effective for your unique needs or diagnose your particular medical history.

About the Author

Amy Adams is a nutritionist and lover of ALL things healthy. You will find her practicing yoga every morning and attending Pilates classes twice a week. She loves cooking and only ever uses natural non-processed ingredients. She was taught to use natural and herbal remedies by her mother who doesn't agree with using antibiotics for common ailments.

Amy has another book published about the miracle substance and uses for honey. Honey: The Natural Miracle Healing Substance

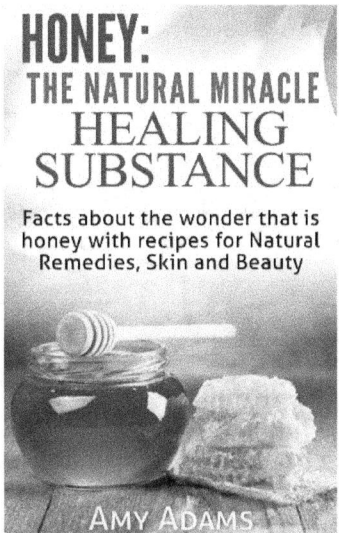

Table of Contents

Introduction

When one of your family members falls ill, what is the first thing you do? You probably pay a visit to your family doctor and, depending on the nature of the ailment, your doctor may prescribe a round of antibiotics. What you may not realize is that the very medicine your doctor gives you feel better may actually have a negative impact on your health. The same antibiotics that are designed to kill harmful bacteria can also come with nasty side effects including upset stomach, diarrhea, vomiting, or skin rash. Are you willing to take the risk that something designed to make you feel better could actually make you feel worse?

If you are concerned about the risks associated with antibiotics, you may be interested to learn that there are a number of natural antibiotic remedies out there. Certain herbs and other natural ingredients have powerful antibiotic properties that can relieve your symptoms quickly and naturally – without a prescription. In this book you will learn the basics about natural herbal antibiotics and receive a collection of recipes to get you started in making your own herbal antibiotics at home.

Chapter One: Antibiotic Resistance and Natural Remedies

In 1954, a total of 2 million pounds of antibiotics were produced and sold. By the year 2000, that number had exploded to 54 million. It is estimated that up to 80% of the antibiotics prescribed for certain conditions such as upper respiratory infections are unnecessary. The danger of producing and prescribing antibiotics in such large quantities is that the bacteria they are designed to treat will eventually become resistant. The more resistant the bacteria become, the greater their potential to cause serious diseases for which there is no prescription.

What is Antibiotic Resistance?

Antibiotic resistance is the resistance (or immunity) to certain antibiotics that occurs in the bacteria responsible for common diseases and infections such as the common cold and the flu. This is an ever-increasing problem that is now present in all parts of the world, largely the result of overuse and misuse of antibiotics. In 2012, an estimated 450,000 cases of tuberculosis were found to be drug-resistant. Those cases required longer, more extensive treatments that were ultimately less effective than the antibiotics should have been. The more this problem spreads, the greater the risk of serious illness (and even death) from even the most common diseases.

What are the Benefits of Herbal and Natural Treatments?

Natural antibiotics are simply the foods that contain natural antibiotic properties as well as the products made from those foods. Centuries ago, before advances in modern medicine, herbs and plants were the only option when it came to antibiotics – the phytochemicals found in these plants performed the same antibiotic role as modern prescription drugs, without the side effects or risk for antibiotic resistance. In addition to their bactericidal properties, natural antibiotic herbs and plants also help to stimulate the immune system while providing anti-inflammatory and anti-septic properties which both kill and inhibit the growth of bacteria. In short, herbal and natural antibiotic treatments are just as effective as prescription drugs without the negative side effects and, because they are all-natural, they can work against even the most drug-resistant bacteria.

Chapter Two: Antibiotic Herbs

While prescription antibiotics have the potential to do more harm than good, there are plenty of herbs that offer natural antibiotic benefits. In this chapter you will find a list of the top 12 herbs with natural antibiotic properties. After learning the benefits of these antibiotic herbs, you will receive a collection of homemade antibiotic remedies in the next chapter.

The Top 12 Natural Antibiotic Herbs Include:

Basil	Ginger
Calendula	Mullein
Cinnamon	Myrrh
Clove	Oregon Grape Root
Echinacea	Sage
Garlic	Thyme

Basil

Basil is a fragrant herb, the leaves of which can be used to create a variety of herbal remedies. This herb has both antibacterial and antimicrobial properties that are most heavily concentrated in its essential oil. Basil has been used to treat stomach spasms, gas, fluid retention, head colds, warts, and worm infections – when applied topically, it can also help to treat insect bites and snake bites.

Calendula

Calendula is a flowering herb, the flowers of which can be used to create antibacterial remedies. This herb has been used to treat sore throat, menstrual cramps, and stomach ulcers – it has also been used to prevent muscle spasms and to reduce fever. When applied directly to the skin, calendula can be used to treat ulcers, poorly healing wounds, inflammation, and varicose veins.

Cinnamon

Cinnamon is a fragrant spice derived from the bark of the cinnamon tree. This spice has been used to treat upset stomach, diarrhea, gas, menstrual cramps, cold and flu – it is also very effective against bacteria and parasitic worms. When applied to the skin, the essential oils in cinnamon have been shown to increase blood flow and to reduce spasms.

Clove

Clove is an herb and its flower buds, leaves, and stems can be used in a variety of antibacterial and herbal remedies. The essential oil of clove is particularly beneficial as a topical analgesic and as a treatment for intestinal bacteria. Clove has also been used to treat upset stomach, nausea, diarrhea, and vomiting.

Echinacea

The flowers, leaves, and roots of the Echinacea herb are widely used to treat the common cold and various other infections including upper respiratory infection. When taken at the first sign of a cold, Echinacea has been shown to help reduce the duration and severity of the illness. Echinacea has also been used to treat flu, urinary tract infections, yeast infections, septicemia, strep throat, and various other infections. When applied topically, Echinacea can help to treat boils, abscesses, skin wounds, burns, eczema, psoriasis, bee stings, and hemorrhoids.

Garlic

The health benefits of garlic are vast and varied, though its antibacterial qualities are not to be overlooked. This herb has been proven to be more effective against certain types of bacteria than even penicillin – it is also gentler on the body because it doesn't affect the body's natural gut flora. Garlic can be used to treat fever, cough, headache, stomach ache, gout, asthma, and bronchitis as well as various fungal infections of the skin including ringworm and athlete's foot.

Ginger

Ginger root contains a number of powerful active ingredients including gingerols, zingerone, and shogaol – these active ingredients are closely linked to ginger's antibacterial benefits. Ginger is also a powerful anti-inflammatory agent as well as a pain reliever. This herb can be used to treat stomach aches, morning sickness, gas, diarrhea, and vomiting. It can also be applied to the skin as a treatment for burns.

Mullein

Mullein is a very gentle herb which makes it the perfect natural antibiotic remedy for children. This herb has traditionally been used to treat coughs, sore throat, headache, fever, flu, earache, cold, and pneumonia. It can also be applied to the skin as a treatment for wounds, burns, bruises, frostbite, and skin infections.

Myrrh

Though it is not technically an herb, myrrh is derived from a plant and it has been used for centuries as a natural antibiotic and herbal remedy. Myrrh is a sap that can be used to create herbal remedies for cold, cough, indigestion, ulcers and asthma. It can also be directly applied to the skin as a treatment for wounds, boils and abrasions, or to the mouth for chapped lips, inflamed gums, or gingivitis.

Oregon Grape Root

The root of the Oregon grape plant can be used to create herbal remedies for a variety of conditions including stomach ulcers, upset stomach, systemic infections, and gastroesophageal reflux disease (GERD). When applied directly to the skin, Oregano grape root acts as a disinfectant and as a powerful treatment for psoriasis.

Sage

Sage is a fragrant herb, the leaves of which can be used to make natural antibiotics and herbal remedies. This herb has been used to treat gas, stomach pain, diarrhea, and digestive upset – it has also been used as a treatment for depression and memory loss.

When applied directly to the skin, sage can help treat cold sores, gum disease, sore throat, and swelling.

Thyme

The flowers, leaves, and essential oil of the thyme plant offer strong antibacterial benefits. This herb has been used to treat various respiratory conditions including bronchitis, whooping cough, and sore throat as well as colic, arthritis, stomach pain, diarrhea, and flatulence. When applies directly to the skin, thyme can also help to treat baldness, ear infection, hoarseness, and swollen tonsils.

Chapter Three: Natural Antibiotic Recipes

Recipes Included in this Book:

Basic Antibiotic Ointment   Oregon Grape Ointment for Psoriasis

Flu-Fighting Tea   Ginger Turmeric Tea

Thyme Tea for Cough   Marshmallow Root Tea for Heartburn

Wound-Healing Clay   Sage Tea for Sore Throat

Echinacea Tincture   Myrrh Salve for Arthritis

Calendula Salve for Eczema   Multi-Use Garlic Infusion

DIY Diaper Rash Cream   Fever-Reducing Basil Infusion

Immuno-Boosting Tincture   Clove Compress for Toothache

Cinnamon Lemon Cough Syrup   Garlic Mullein Earache Treatment

Basic Antibiotic Ointment

This basic antibiotic ointment is the perfect all-purpose ointment to have on hand for cuts, scrapes, and burns. Apply this ointment as you would a commercial antibiotic ointment like Neosporin and cover with a clean bandage or gauze.

Ingredients:

1 tablespoon beeswax, grated

1 ounce jojoba oil

1 ounce sweet almond oil

6 drops peppermint essential oil

5 drops lavender essential oil

5 drops tea tree essential oil

Instructions:

1. Melt the beeswax, jojoba oil, and almond oil in a double boiler over low heat.
2. Stir well until thoroughly combined then remove from heat.
3. Allow the mixture to cool to room temperature then stir in the essential oils.
4. Pour the mixture into the glass jar and cover tightly with the lid.
5. Apply to clean, dry skin as an antibiotic ointment.

Flu-Fighting Tea

This herbal antibiotic tea is easy to throw together when you feel a cold or flu coming on. Not only does it help to boost your immune system, but the cayenne will warm your body, helping you to sweat out toxins. Both honey and garlic are natural antibiotics which will help you to fight the illness while also soothing a sore throat.

Ingredients:

Small glass jar

½ cup fresh lemon juice

2 tablespoons Manuka honey

2 tablespoons fresh minced ginger

½ teaspoon ground cinnamon

¼ teaspoon ground cayenne

1 clove garlic, crushed

Instructions:

1. Pour the lemon juice into the glass jar.
2. Stir in the remaining ingredients until thoroughly combined.
3. Take 1 tablespoon of the mixture in 6 to 8 ounces hot water 2 to 3 times daily as needed.
4. If you are not drinking the tea immediately, omit the garlic until you are ready to take it – refrigerate up to 2 days.

Wound-Healing Clay

Medicinal clay has been used for centuries to heal all manner of physical conditions including cuts, scrapes, sprains, insect bites, burns, and more. This wound-healing clay can be combined with water to form a paste that you will then spread on the afflicted area to soothe and heal.

Ingredients:

½ cup powdered green clay

2 tablespoons Oregon grape root powder

2 tablespoons aloe vera powder

2 tablespoons comfrey root powder

Small glass jar

Water

Instructions:

1. Combine the green clay, Oregon grape root powder, aloe vera powder, and comfrey root powder in a small glass jar.
2. Stir the mixture until thoroughly combined and cover tightly with the lid.
3. When ready to use, spoon a small amount of powder into your hand and mix with a few drops of water to form a paste.
4. Spread the paste on the afflicted area to soothe and heal.

Thyme Tea for Cough

Thyme is known for its natural antibacterial properties and for being a strong herbal remedy for a variety of respiratory conditions. In this tea, the thyme acts as a powerful expectorant while the honey soothes and the ginger heals.

Ingredients:

1 cup boiling water

2 tablespoons dried thyme

½ to 1 tablespoon Manuka honey

1 tablespoon fresh lemon juice

1 teaspoon fresh grated ginger

½ teaspoon ground turmeric

Pinch cayenne

Instructions:

1. Steep the thyme in a cup of boiling water for 10 minutes.
2. Strain out the thyme then stir in the remaining ingredients.
3. Drink immediately to soothe and relieve cough 3 to 4 times a day.

Echinacea Tincture

Echinacea is a natural antibiotic herb that has a number of health benefits. Not only can it help to stave off colds and flu, but it can also be used to soothe sore throats, respiratory infections, and even strep throat. This is one tincture that you will want to keep on hand during flu season.

Ingredients:

2 cups high-proof vodka

¼ cup dried Echinacea, crushed

Glass pint jar

Instructions:

1. Place the Echinacea in the pint jar and pour in the vodka, leaving a little room for air at the top of the jar.
2. Cover tightly with the lid and label the jar.
3. Let the tincture sit at room temperature for 4 to 6 weeks, shaking every few days.
4. Strain the Echinacea out of the vodka using a piece of fine mesh or cheesecloth.
5. Return the liquid to the jar and store in a dark, cool place.
6. To use, take ½ to ¾ teaspoon of the tincture directly under the tongue 3 to 4 times daily when you feel a cold coming on.

Calendula Salve for Eczema

The flowers of the calendula plant have been known to heal a wide variety of skin conditions including eczema and psoriasis. In this recipe, calendula flowers are combined with bees wax and olive oil for their moisturizing benefits to create a soothing and healing salve.

Ingredients:

¾ cups extra-virgin olive oil

½ cup dried calendula flowers

2 tablespoons beeswax

Small glass jar, with lid

Pot of boiling water

Instructions:

1. Bring several inches of water to boil in a saucepot or skillet.
2. Place the calendula flowers in the glass jar and pour in the olive oil.
3. Put the jar in the boiling water – remove water, if needed, to ensure that no water gets into the jar.
4. Reduce the heat to a simmer and warm the jar for 4 to 5 hours, adding water as needed.
5. Remove the pan from the heat and take the jar out of the water.
6. Strain the liquid from the jar through a mesh strainer and discard the calendula flowers – squeeze as much oil as possible from them.
7. Pour the liquid back into the jar and add the beeswax.
8. Place the jar back in the water to melt the beeswax – stir occasionally until the wax is melted and thoroughly incorporated.
9. Remove from heat and allow the salve to cool to room temperature.
10. Spread the salve on irritated skin to treat eczema, psoriasis, cuts, scrapes, and burns.

DIY Diaper Rash Cream

This DIY diaper rash cream is simple to throw together and highly effective. The shea butter helps to moisturize your baby's skin while the calendula heals the skin. Lavender oil has antibacterial properties which helps to cure the rash and coconut oil soothes.

Ingredients:

Small glass jar (with lid)

2 ounces water

1 ounce sweet almond oil

2 tablespoons dried calendula flowers

1 tablespoon shea butter

1 tablespoon coconut oil

1 tablespoon beeswax

8 drops lavender essential oil

Instructions:

1. Combine the water and calendula flowers in a small saucepan.
2. Bring to a simmer and simmer for 10 to 15 minutes.
3. Strain the mixture, reserving the liquid. Set aside.
4. In a double boiler, melt together the shea butter, beeswax, coconut oil, and sweet almond oil.
5. Stir in 2 tablespoons of the reserved liquid along with the lavender essential oil.
6. Pour the mixture into the glass jar and allow to cool completely.
7. Spread the cream on irritated skin to relieve and heal diaper rash.

Immuno-Boosting Tincture

This tincture is made from a variety of herbs that are known not only for their antibiotic properties but also for their healing, and restorative benefits. Use this tincture to boost your immune system when you feel a cold coming on or to help soothe a sore throat or cough when you are already sick.

Ingredients:

½ cup dried mullein, leaves and flowers

¼ cup dried spearmint, crushed

¼ cup dried yarrow leaf, crushed

2 tablespoons dried lemon balm, crushed

1/3 cup vegetable glycerin (food grade)

1/3 cup water

Instructions:

1. Combine the dried herbs in a glass pint jar.
2. Pour in the glycerin and stir gently to combine.
3. Add the water, stirring until everything is thoroughly combined and the dried herbs are completely saturated.
4. Put the lid on the jar and let it sit at room temperature for 6 weeks.
5. After 6 weeks, strain the mixture through a piece of fine mesh or cheesecloth and return the liquid to the jar.
6. Take 1 teaspoon of the tincture directly under the tongue two to three times a day as needed.

Cinnamon Lemon Cough Syrup

This homemade antibiotic remedy for cough is incredibly easy to prepare and it tastes better than anything you would buy at the store. Both cinnamon and honey are known for their antibacterial qualities and, in this recipe, the honey coats your throat, soothing and relieving soreness from cough.

Ingredients:

1 cup water

1 cup Manuka honey

½ cup fresh lemon juice

1 tablespoon fresh lemon zest

2 tablespoons fresh grated ginger

1 tablespoon ground cinnamon

Instructions:

1. Combine the water, lemon zest and ginger in a small saucepot.
2. Bring the mixture to a boil then reduce heat and simmer for 5 minutes.
3. Strain the mixture into a glass jar and discard the solids.
4. Pour the honey into the saucepan and warm on low heat for 5 minutes.
5. Stir in the lemon juice, cinnamon and reserved liquid.
6. Whisk until the mixture forms a thick syrup then pour into the glass jar.
7. Cover tightly with the lid and refrigerate for up to 2 months.
8. Take 1 to 2 tablespoons every four hours for adults.
9. For children aged 5 to 12, take 1 to 2 teaspoons every 2 hours.

Oregon Grape Ointment for Psoriasis

When taken internally, Oregon grape root is a powerful antibiotic treatment for stomach problems but, when applied topically, it is a great remedy for psoriasis and other skin problems. Oregon grape root contains natural tannins that reduce the formation of certain types of skin cells which is why it is so powerful against the inflammation and irritation caused by psoriasis.

Ingredients:

1 tablespoon dried calendula flowers, crushed

½ tablespoon dried Oregon grape root, crushed

½ tablespoon dried St. John's wort, crushed

2 to 3 ounces beeswax, grated

Glass jar, with lid

Metal tin, with lid

Instructions:

1. Combine the herbs in the glass jar and pour in the olive oil.
2. Stir well to combine then let sit at room temperature for 4 to 6 weeks to form a tincture.
3. Strain the mixture through a piece of fine mesh or cheesecloth, squeezing as much oil from the herbs as possible.
4. Pour the oil into a glass jar and discard the solids – you should have at least 1 cup of oil.
5. Melt the beeswax in a small saucepan over low heat.
6. Remove from heat and stir in the oil until it is thoroughly combined.
7. Pour the ointment into a metal tin then cover tightly with the lid and store at room temperature.
8. Apply the ointment to clean, dry skin to soothe and heal psoriasis.

Ginger Turmeric Tea

Both ginger and turmeric contain natural anti-inflammatory properties which helps to soothe and relieve arthritis and other types of joint pain. The active ingredient in these spices is curcumin, a powerful antioxidant. Enjoy this tea twice daily to relieve the symptoms of arthritis – feel free to sweeten it with honey.

Ingredients:

1 cup water

¼ teaspoon ground ginger

¼ teaspoon ground turmeric

Honey to taste

Instructions:

1. Bring the water to boil in a small saucepan.
2. Stir in the ginger and turmeric then simmer for 10 to 15 minutes.
3. Strain the mixture through a piece of fine mesh or cheesecloth into a mug.
4. Sweeten with honey to taste and enjoy immediately.

Marshmallow Root Tea for Heartburn

Marshmallow root is an herb that contains mucilage – this substance has been shown to coat the esophagus, soothing inflammation and irritation from acid reflux and heartburn. This marshmallow root tea is easy to prepare and should be taken 1 to 3 times per day as a treatment for heartburn.

Ingredients:

1 tablespoon dried marshmallow root

8 ounces boiling water

Honey to sweeten, optional

Instructions:

1. Steep the marshmallow root in 8 ounces of boiling water for 10 minutes.
2. Strain the mixture through a piece of fine mesh or cheesecloth and discard the solids.
3. Pour the liquid into a tea cup or mug and enjoy immediately.
4. Drink this tea up to three times daily as a treatment for heartburn.

Sage Tea for Sore Throat

Sage is known for providing a wide variety of medicinal benefits, not the least of which is soothing sore throats. The tannins in sage also help to stimulate digestive secretions which improves your body's resistance to infection. Enjoy this tea up to two times daily to soothe a sore throat or use it as a warm gargle.

Ingredients:

1 cup boiling water

1 teaspoon dried sage, crushed

½ teaspoon fennel seeds

Instructions:

1. Place the sage and fennel in a mug.
2. Pour the boiling water over the ingredients and let steep for 5 minutes or until it reaches the desired strength.
3. Strain the mixture through fine mesh or cheesecloth and discard the solids.
4. Sweeten the tea with honey, if desired, and enjoy 1 to 2 times daily.

Myrrh Salve for Arthritis

Myrrh essential oil not only helps to soothe pain and inflammation from arthritis, but it can also relax the spirit and help to speed healing. Use this salve to soothe sore and inflamed joints as an alternative to over-the-counter or prescription arthritis medications.

Ingredients:

¾ cups extra-virgin olive oil

½ cup dried thyme, crushed

2 tablespoons beeswax

10 drops myrrh essential oil

Small glass jar, with lid

Pot of boiling water

Instructions:

1. Bring several inches of water to boil in a saucepot or skillet.
2. Place the thyme in the glass jar and pour in the olive oil.
3. Put the jar in the boiling water – remove water, if needed, to ensure that no water gets into the jar.
4. Reduce the heat to a simmer and warm the jar for 4 to 5 hours, adding water as needed.
5. Remove the pan from the heat and take the jar out of the water.
6. Strain the liquid from the jar through a mesh strainer and discard the thyme.
7. Pour the liquid back into the jar and add the beeswax and myrrh essential oil.
8. Place the jar back in the water to melt the beeswax – stir occasionally until the wax is melted and thoroughly incorporated.
9. Remove from heat and allow the salve to cool to room temperature.
10. Rub the salve into the skin over sore joints to soothe and relieve inflammation.

Multi-Use Garlic Infusion

Garlic is widely known for its antibacterial and antioxidant power. This garlic infusion can be used for a wide variety of purposes – use it as an antiseptic to treat yeast infections or as a general antibiotic to protect your body against various diseases. The best part about this infusion is that it will help destroy pathogenic bacteria while preserving the good bacteria in your digestive system.

Ingredients:

½ cup fresh minced garlic

¾ cup extra-virgin olive oil

Instructions:

1. Combine the garlic and olive oil in a glass jar and cover tightly with the lid.
2. Let the mixture sit in a warm, sunny area for 2 weeks to infuse, shaking the jar 2 to 3 times per day.
3. Strain the mixture through a piece of fine mesh or cheesecloth and discard the solids.
4. Store the infusion in a glass jar in the refrigerator.
5. Take 1 teaspoon of the infusion in 5 ounces of water daily.

Fever-Reducing Basil Infusion

Basil is a fragrant herb that is known for providing a wide variety of medicinal benefits. In this recipe, basil helps to cool and reduce fever. Sip this infusion slowly when you first notice the fever and expect relief to occur within the next few hours. Feel free to add more honey to sweeten the infusion.

Ingredients:

4 fresh basil leaves

1 cup boiling water

½ cup organic milk

1 to 2 teaspoons Manuka honey

¼ teaspoon ground cardamom

Instructions:

1. Place the basil leaves in a mug and pour in the boiling water.
2. Let the leaves steep for 5 to 10 minutes then strain the liquid to remove the leaves.
3. Pour the liquid back into the mug and slowly stir in the milk, honey, and ground cardamom.
4. Sip the tea slowly to reduce fever.

Clove Compress for Toothache

Toothaches can occur for a wide variety of reasons and they can be both painful and difficult to treat. Rather than taking a general pain reliever like ibuprofen, bring pain relief directly to the affected area with this clove compress. While this compress will not treat the cause of the toothache, it will bring you relief from pain.

Ingredients:

Warm saltwater

½ teaspoon olive oil

3 drops clove essential oil

Clean cotton balls

Instructions:

1. Gargle warm saltwater to clean your mouth before applying the compress.
2. Combine the clove essential oil and olive oil in a small bowl – stir well.
3. Soak a cotton ball in the mixture then press it firmly against the sore tooth.

Garlic Mullein Earache Treatment

Earaches are a common malady that tend to affect young children and they can be incredibly painful. Rather than treating your child with an over-the-counter medication that could cause side effects, try this natural remedy made with garlic and mullein. Garlic is a powerful antibiotic that can help to treat the infection and mullein helps to soothe the pain in a way that is gentle enough for children.

Ingredients:

¼ cup extra virgin olive oil

½ cup dried mullein, crushed

4 cloves garlic, crushed

Instructions:

1. Warm the oil in a small saucepan over medium-low heat.
2. Stir in the garlic and mullein until fully saturated with oil.
3. Let the mixture simmer on low heat for 1 to 2 hours – be careful that it doesn't burn.
4. Strain the mixture through a piece of fine mesh or cheesecloth and discard the solids.
5. Pour the oil into a dark colored bottle and store in a cool, dry place.
6. To use, warm the bottle of oil in a cup of hot water and apply a few drops to the affected ear to reduce pain.

Conclusion

After reading this book you should have a good idea what antibiotic resistance is and how natural antibiotics and herbal remedies are better for your body than prescription antibiotics. In addition to receiving basic information about herbal antibiotics, you also received a detailed overview of the top 12 antibacterial herbs as well as a list of conditions they can be used to treat. Finally, you received a collection of natural antibiotic and herbal remedies for common conditions including cold, flu, skin infections, and so much more.